Copyright ©2023.

Table of Contents

Introduction

The alkaline diet is based on the claim that eating foods with a higher pH, or those that are more alkaline, will help reduce your risk of chronic diseases like cancer. Although alkaline diets as a form of dietary therapy began in the twentieth century, the science underlying research into the body's pH balance began in nineteenth-century France. A bomb calorimeter consists of a chamber with pressurized oxygen suspended in a water bath. The food to be tested is placed in the chamber and ignited by an electric current. The pressurized oxygen ensures that the food is combusted rapidly and completely. The ash that remains can then be mixed with pure water and tested to determine its acidity or alkalinity. Consequently, the effect of alkaline-ash foods in lowering the acidity of urine was studied as a possible way to prevent kidney stone formation and/or lower the risk of urinary tract infections. This was the original purpose of alkaline diets; however, they were rapidly superseded by drug therapy for kidney stones and UTIs because of the difficulty of making precise calculations of the effects of food on urinary pH. As of 2018, the level of detail and precision needed to make such calculations is still formidable, as samples of specific foods not only vary somewhat in their acidity, but human's also vary in their rate of absorption of the nutrients in food. The third stage in the development of alkaline diets was an unwarranted assumption on the part of some alternative medicine practitioner that alkaline-ash foods can affect the pH of the body in general and blood in particular, not just the urine. This assumption is not supported by the actual mechanism of acid-base homeostasis, which maintains the pH of human blood as slightly alkaline within a narrow range between 7.35 and 7.45. Levels above 7.45 lead to a condition called alkalosis; levels below 7.45 lead to acidosis. Both are potentially serious conditions. In healthy humans, acid-base homeostasis is maintained by the respiratory system and the urinary system, neither of which is controlled by dietary intake. The alkaline diet, also called the alkaline ash diet or alkaline acid diet, was made popular by its celebrity followers.

What Is the Alkaline Diet Exactly?

Definition

Alkaline diets are a group of diets based on the discredited notion that the body's pH balance (its relative acidity or alkalinity) can be affected by the dieter's choice of foods. Proponents of alkaline diets hold that eating meats, fish, dairy products, and other high-protein foods increases the body's acidity and thereby increases the risk of cancer, heart disease, bone loss, other chronic disorders, and low energy levels. Alkaline diets are also known as acid alkaline diets, alkaline acid diets, alkaline ash diets, and acid ash diets. The word ash in this context refers to the solid material left when a food is completely combusted in a bomb calorimeter, not to the ashes left by a wood or charcoal fire.

Description

There is no single alkaline diet, which can be confusing to consumers. Some so-called alkaline diets are short-term cleansing diets based on fruit and vegetable juice, whereas others are longer-term plans in which dieter's add a higher proportion of alkaline-ash foods to their eating plan. No standard has been established for the ratio of alkaline-ash to acidic-ash foods recommended by these diets. Although an 80/20 ratio is the figure most commonly given, some diets recommend a 60/40 ratio. Alkaline diets are essentially a matter of food selection rather than calorie counting or portion weighing.

Most alkaline diets divide foods into alkaline and acidic categories as follows:

Alkaline foods:

- Fruits: blackcurrants, apples, oranges, apricots, peaches, pears, watermelon, strawberries, raisins
- Vegetables: tomatoes, celery, carrots, asparagus, broccoli, cucumbers, green beans, lettuce, spinach, potatoes.
- Legumes: soybeans, tofu
- Beverages: unsweetened apple juice
- Sweeteners: honey

Acidic foods:

- Meats: chicken, pork, beef, turkey, salami
- Fish: cod, trout
- Eggs and Dairy: eggs, whole milk, ice cream, cheese, cottage cheese, yogurt
- Legumes: lentils
- Nuts: walnuts, peanuts
- Grain products: white bread, whole wheat bread, brown rice, pasta, white flour
- Beverages: coffee, alcoholic beverages
- Ultraprocessed foods

Some versions of the alkaline diet have different lists of "forbidden" foods, though most include processed foods, caffeinated beverages, refined sugar, and alcohol as foods to be avoided.

Alkaline diets do not usually contain any recommendations about physical exercise. In addition, some websites that offer information about these diets also encourage viewers to purchase dietary supplements, books or online courses, and alkaline water or alkaline infused foods. It is not necessary to use any of these items to follow an alkaline diet. Moreover, the U.S. Food and Drug Administration (FDA) has sent recall notices since the early 2000s to manufacturers whose alkaline water products were misbranded and has denied the health claims (specifically, that these products can prevent osteoporosis) of alkaline products distributed by other manufacturers. These health claims were based on a debate in the medical literature in the early 2000s about the possible role of alkaline water in preventing bone loss.

Function

Despite the fact that consumption of alkaline-ash foods does not affect the pH of the blood or body tissues, alkaline diets have been recommended, primarily by naturopaths and other practitioners of alternative medicine, for a variety of reasons ranging from losing weight and slowing the aging process to preventing osteoporosis, kidney stones, cancer, headaches, and the common cold. Alkaline diets are also touted for boosting energy.

Benefits

Most people who follow an alkaline diet will lose weight, at least initially, because the fruits and vegetables identified as alkaline contain less fat and fewer calories than the meats, grain products, and dairy products categorized as acidic. In addition, alkaline diets are compatible with vegetarian and vegan lifestyles. A third benefit is that alkaline diets are generally easier on the budget than food plans that allow meat, dairy products, and sweets.

Some people who have tried alkaline diets find them more effective than other weight loss diets in managing hunger because the permitted foods are relatively filling due to their bulk and fiber content, and no limits are set on portion size.

Precautions

People diagnosed with cancer should consult their physician or a dietitian about their nutritional needs before starting any kind of diet. People taking medications for osteoporosis, arthritis, urinary tract infections, kidney stones, headaches, or other conditions supposedly treated by alkaline diets should not stop taking their medications if they decide to try an alkaline diet.

People who follow an alkaline diet plan must be careful to obtain enough protein and calcium from the foods they do consume because many sources of protein and calcium allowed in moderation in other diets, such as lean meat or skim milk, are not allowed in alkaline diet plans.

Many people find alkaline diets difficult to follow not only because of the restricted number of foods permitted but also because these diets complicate eating out or sharing a household with family members who do not follow the diet. In addition, alkaline diets frequently add to the time and labor involved in food preparation because processed foods are not allowed.

Long-term use of an alkaline diet puts the dieter at risk of nutritional deficiencies resulting from low intake of calcium, protein, and essential fatty acids. In addition, people who stop the use of medications prescribed to treat such disorders as arthritis, cancer, diabetes, osteoporosis, or kidney stones because they believe that an alkaline diet is sufficient treatment for their condition are at risk of having their symptoms worsen.

Dieters who purchase alkaline water or other alkaline supplements to accompany the diet are at risk of being defrauded by manufacturers who misbrand their products or make unproven health claims. In addition, the FDA notes that some samples of socalled alkaline water have been found to be contaminated by salmonella and other bacteria.

Research and General Acceptance

People interested in an alkaline diet should be aware that medical and nutrition professionals as well as many naturopaths dismiss these diets as fad diets. It is significant that neither the Academy of Nutrition and Dietetics (AND) nor the National Center for Complementary and Integrative Health (NCCIH) even mentions alkaline diets on their websites. In regard to naturopathy, responsible practitioners point out that the theory underlying alkaline diets is contrary to everything known about the chemistry of the human body, even though the overall results of a diet high in fruits and vegetables and low in fats and refined sugar are beneficial in regard to weight loss and heart health. Alkaline diets also scored low on the U.S. News and World Report Health rating (2.4 out of a possible 5) because of their many arbitrary rules about food choices and because they have been poorly researched.

As of 2018, few mainstream clinical trials have been conducted of either alkaline diets or alkaline water and other dietary supplements. Four studies of alkaline water had been registered with the

National Institutes of Health as of early 2018. One was a study of alkaline water as a sports beverage; another was looking at whether alkaline water reduces skin toxicity in women being treated with radiation therapy for breast cancer. The remaining two were studies of the effect of alkaline water on the pH of human urine.

Though there is no research to support these claims, the premise of the alkaline diet is that the foods you eat can change your body's pH. Promoters of the diet believe that by eating foods that are less acidic and more alkaline, you'll be protected from several health issues.

Key Terms

Acid-Ash hypothesis

A outdated medical theory that attributed osteoporosis and other negative health effects to excessively acidic diets. The theory held that meat, poultry, fish, and other high-protein foods that produce acidic ash after combustion induce the body to reduce the level of acid by removing calcium from bone, thus weakening bone and increasing the risk of osteoporosis.

Acid-Base Homeostasis

The regulation of the pH of the body's extracellular fluid (ECF) at a stable level. Extracellular fluid accounts for about a third of the human body's total water content.

Ash

In analytical chemistry, the nonliquid and nongaseous residue left after the complete combustion of a substance. Reducing a substance to ash is done to analyze and measure its metal and mineral content.

Bomb Calorimeter

A type of constant-volume device used to measure the amount of heat produced by combustion of a specific substance. Bomb calorimeters are often used to measure the calorie content of foods.

Legume

Any plant belonging to the family Fabaceae. Legumes are grown for their grain seeds and for livestock forage; they include chickpeas, alfalfa, lentils, clover, peas, beans, soybeans, and peanuts.

Naturopathy

A system of disease treatment that emphasizes natural means of health care, such as water, natural foods, herbs and other dietary adjustments, massage and manipulation, and electrotherapy, and rather than conventional drugs and surgery.

PH

A numeric scale used in chemistry to denote the acidity or alkalinity of an aqueous (water-based) solution. Solutions with numbers below 7 are acid; those with numbers above 7 are alkaline. Pure water has a pH of 7 and is neutral.

Tofu

Bean curd; a soft food made by coagulating soymilk with an enzyme, calcium sulfate, or an organic acid, and pressing the resulting curds into blocks or chunks. Tofu is frequently used in vegetarian or vegan dishes as a meat or cheese substitute.

How Does the Plan Work?

The alkaline diet emphasizes consuming alkaline foods in an attempt to make the body's pH more alkaline. That said, it is impossible to change the body's pH through diet. Indeed, the body's pH actually varies based on the region. For example, the stomach is more acidic. (More on this later.)

Is This How Our Ancestors Ate?

The alkaline diet's emphasis on fruit and vegetables over processed foods overlaps considerably with the paleo diet, which is meant to mimic the dietary habits of our hunter-and-gatherer ancestors. But research doesn't necessarily support the idea that our early ancestors consumed alkaline diets. According to previous research, about one-half of the 229 historical diets researchers of the paper looked at were acid-producing, while the other half were alkaline-forming.

Another past study found the disparity may be location-based. The researchers found that the farther away from the equator that people lived, the more acidic their diets were. Because ancestors of Homo sapiens lived in East Africa, which is closer to the equator, they were likely following alkaline diets.

More on What Studies Suggest About Food and pH

The kidneys and lungs are largely responsible for maintaining a balanced pH in the body, and it's very tightly regulated. Blood pH ranges from 7.2 to 7.45, says Jennifer Fitzgibbon, RDN, a registered oncology dietitian at Stony Brook University Cancer Center in New York. The kidneys also help balance pH levels in urine, according to UC San Diego Health. A urine pH of 4 is considered strongly acidic, while 7 is neutral and 9 is strongly alkaline, notes Michigan Medicine.

What's the Difference Between Ketosis and Diabetic Ketoacidosis?

But here's the tricky part: A style of eating can't change your body's pH. You may notice a difference in your urine pH, which can be measured with a simple dipstick test (also called a urine test strip), but that won't tell you your overall levels because urine pH doesn't reflect your body's pH, according to MedlinePlus. That's because excess acid might be excreted through the urine in order to balance the body's pH levels, notes the American Institute for Cancer Research.

If your body's pH changes, it is because of a serious health issue. Urine with a high pH could indicate a urinary tract infection (UTI) or kidney stones, while a low pH could signify diarrhea, starvation, or diabetic ketoacidosis.

Reduced Risk of Cancer, and Other Benefits?

Advocates of the alkaline diet make some bold claims. The primary focus of the eating approach isn't weight loss — although that's a likely result given the restrictions — but instead disease prevention and treatment. Followers and authors of the many guides and recipe books say the alkaline diet can treat diseases and chronic conditions, including cancer and kidney disease.

From a scientific perspective, these claims aren't realistic, says Adrienne Youdim, MD, an associate professor of medicine at the UCLA David Geffen School of Medicine in Los Angeles. But, she says, the foods listed as alkaline tend to be healthy, and when you look at eating approaches like the widely studied and beneficial Mediterranean diet, you can reasonably say the focus on these foods is a healthy approach.

Who Is the Alkaline Diet Best For?

A more relaxed version of the alkaline diet that doesn't strictly eliminate healthy nuts and grains can be beneficial for overall health. Fundamentally, a plant-based diet can be good for lowering your risk of many cancers, heart disease, type 2 diabetes, and stroke, notes the American Heart Association. For those with a history of kidney stones or kidney disease, a plant-based diet — but not necessarily an alkaline diet — may help.

Who Should Avoid the Alkaline Diet?

For people without preexisting health conditions, the alkaline diet is generally safe, but some people may be left feeling hungry or may not get enough protein for their needs. In addition to restricting many unhealthy foods, some healthy foods are left out as well.

Although the focus is on healthy plant-based foods, the alkaline diet is not designed for weight loss, and there are no guides for portion control or fitness routines, which the Centers for Disease Control and Prevention recommends for disease prevention.

Also, if you aren't sure how to get enough protein using plant sources, you could be left feeling very hungry.

What Else to Know Before Trying the Alkaline Diet

In any case, you should talk with your healthcare team before trying the alkaline diet. Because the eating approach can be restrictive, you want to make sure you're not cutting out important nutrients or unintentionally harming your health.

Is It Good for Certain Conditions?

Following an alkaline diet means choosing fruits and vegetables over higher-calorie, higher-fat choices. You will also shun prepared foods, which often have a lot of sodium.

That's great news for heart health because these steps help lower blood pressure and cholesterol, which are big risk factors for heart disease.

Getting to a healthy weight is also important in preventing and treating diabetes and osteoarthritis.

Some studies have found that an alkaline environment may make certain chemotherapy drugs more effective or less toxic. But it has not been shown that an alkaline diet can do this or help prevent cancer. If you have cancer, talk to your doctor or dietitian about your nutritional needs before starting any type of diet.

How does the Alkaline Diet Support You?

If you're looking to start the acid alkaline diet or have already begun your dieting journey, it's helpful to know the different ways you can receive support throughout the process. Below are a few examples of how the acid alkaline diet can support you:

Guidebooks like "Acid Alkaline Diet for Dummies" include extensive lists of alkaline- and acid-forming foods.

How much does Alkaline Diet cost?

Other than your grocery bill, which should be no higher than usual, there are no expenses.

Will Alkaline Diet help you lose weight?

The Alkaline diet will probably help you lose weight. While the Alkaline diet lacks robust clinical studies examining its weight loss potential, its ban on processed food and emphasis on eating whole grains, vegetables and soy products will likely yield weight loss. Just build in a "calorie deficit" – eat fewer calories than your daily recommended max, or burn off extra by exercising – and you should see the numbers on the scale budge. How quickly and whether you keep the weight off, however, is up to you.

The approach also shares tenets with vegetarianism, and vegetarians tend to eat fewer calories and weigh less than their meat-eating counterparts.

How easy is Alkaline Diet to follow?

Adhering to the Alkaline diet takes work. You have to keep track of which foods are alkaline-formers and which are acid-formers. That can be a lot to remember. Recipes are abundant on the internet, but you'll have to put quite a bit of thought into your restaurant meals to make sure they emphasize alkaline-forming foods.

Finding recipes for the Alkaline diet should be easy. A simple Google search yields plenty of options, in addition to several books you can invest in for even more options at your fingertips.

You can eat out on the Alkaline diet, but keep in mind that some restaurants have meals that are more pH-friendly than others. If the menu offers standard American fare, opt for a large salad with just olive oil for dressing, and request steamed veggies in lieu of fries or mashed potatoes. If you're at a Chinese buffet, fill up on veggie- and egg-based soups, steamed broccoli and sauteed chicken or tofu. And if you're going Greek, order a chicken shish kebab – and ditch the hummus and cheese pastries, which are acid-forming.

Planning ahead can help you adhere to the Alkaline diet. But there aren't any timesavers when it comes to following the plan, unless you hire somebody to plan your meals, shop for you and prepare your lunch and dinner. Meal kit delivery services are another option to help cut down on prep time.

Alkaline diet resources are available. Books like "Acid Alkaline Diet for Dummies" can help you get your bearings.

Feeling satisfied probably won't be an issue with this diet. Nutrition experts emphasize the importance of satiety, or the satisfied feeling that you've had enough. With so many fiber-packed whole grains and veggies (and without a calorie cap), you shouldn't go hungry.

Whether the Alkaline diet tastes good is up to you. You're making everything, so if something doesn't taste good, you know who to blame.

How much should you exercise on Alkaline Diet?

The Alkaline Diet is only an eating pattern, but that doesn't mean you shouldn't exercise. Physical activity lowers your risk of heart disease and diabetes, helps keep weight off and increases your energy level. Most experts suggest getting at least 30 minutes of moderate-intensity exercise – like brisk walking – most or all days of the week.

Alkaline Diet Recipes

Diet Soup

There are hundreds of variations, but the main point of the soup is to be full and to get lots of natural fiber. Almost anything can be added or removed to your sense of taste - bell peppers, corn, tomato juice. Try substituting chicken soup mix for the onion soup mix.

Ingredients

1 medium head cabbage, chopped

1 onion, chopped

3 large carrots, chopped

3 stalks celery, chopped

3 tomatoes, chopped

16 ounces frozen green beans

2 (1 ounce) packages dry onion soup mix

6 cups water

Directions

Step 1

Combine water, soup mix, and vegetables in a large stock pot. Bring to a boil. Reduce heat, and simmer until the vegetables are tender.

Nutrition Facts

Per Serving: 94 calories; protein 3.6g; carbohydrates 21g; fat 0.5g; sodium 672.9mg.

Savory Diet Chicken

Very simple, healthy and delicious! The amounts are up to you! (Note: As a general guide, one serving would consist of one chicken breast with 1 to 2 of each of the vegetables). Easy and flexible!

Ingredients

4 skinless, boneless chicken breast halves

6 potatoes

2 green bell peppers, sliced

1 cup cubed carrots

2 onions, quartered

1 dash Worcestershire sauce

1 teaspoon paprika

Directions

Step 1

Preheat oven to 350 degrees F (175 degrees C).

Step 2

In a 9x13 inch baking dish, place the chicken breasts. Add the potatoes, bell peppers, carrot and onion, all cubed or quartered. Sprinkle all liberally with Worcestershire sauce and a dash of paprika.

Cover dish and bake in the preheated oven for 1 1/2 hour. That's it! Enjoy!

Nutrition Facts

Per Serving: 425 calories; protein 35.2g; carbohydrates 67.1g; fat 2.1g; cholesterol 68.4mg; sodium 123mg.

Dash Diet Mexican Bake

Mexican flavors will make this chicken casserole a family favorite.

Ingredients

1½ cups cooked rice, preferably brown

1 pound skinless, boneless chicken breast, cut in bite-sized pieces

2 (14.5 ounce) cans no-salt-added tomatoes, diced or crushed

1 (15 ounce) can no-salt-added black beans, drained and rinsed

1 cup frozen yellow corn kernels

1 cup chopped red bell pepper

1 cup chopped poblano pepper

1 tablespoon chili powder

1 tablespoon cumin

4 garlic cloves, crushed

1 cup shredded reduced-fat Monterey Jack cheese

¼ cup jalapeno pepper slices (Optional)

Directions

Step 1

Preheat oven to 400 degrees. Spread rice in a shallow 3-quart casserole. Top with chicken. In a bowl, combine tomatoes, beans, corn, peppers, seasonings and garlic; pour over chicken. Top with cheese and optional jalapeno. Bake 45 minutes.

Nutrition Facts

Per Serving: 325 calories; protein 28.4g; carbohydrates 36.9g; fat 7.1g; cholesterol 56.5mg; sodium 355.8mg.

Chocolate Chip Cookies for Special Diets

Be sure to use a heat-stable sugar substitute. Since the substitutes vary in strength, use an amount equal to 3/4 cup regular sugar according to the package.

Ingredients

½ cup butter, softened

¾ cup granulated artificial sweetener

2 tablespoons water

½ teaspoon vanilla extract

1 egg, beaten

1 cups all-purpose flour

½ teaspoon baking soda

½ teaspoon salt

½ cup semisweet chocolate chips

½ cup chopped pecans

Directions

Step 1

Preheat oven to 375 degrees F (190 degrees C).

Step 2

In a medium bowl, cream together the butter and sugar substitute. Mix in water, vanilla, and egg. Sift together the flour, baking soda, and salt; stir into the creamed mixture. Mix in the chocolate chips and pecans. Drop cookies by heaping teaspoonfuls onto a cookie sheet.

Step 3

Bake in the preheated oven for 10 to 12 minutes. Remove from cookie sheets to cool on wire racks. These cookies freeze well.

Nutrition Facts

Per Serving: 60 calories; protein 4.2g; carbohydrates 3.5g; fat 3.4g; cholesterol 9mg; sodium 53.8mg.

Keto Diet Low Carb Pancakes

Delicious, easy, and quick keto pancakes. Serve with syrup and customize with your choice of toppings, like pecans, whipped cream, or blueberry jam. If you are strictly Keto, leave out the sugar.

Ingredients

2 ounces cream cheese, softened

2 eggs

1 teaspoon white sugar

½ teaspoon ground cinnamon

Cooking spray

Directions

Step 1

Combine cream cheese, eggs, sugar, and cinnamon in a blender; blend until smooth. Let rest 2 minutes or lightly tap on counter to remove bubbles.

Step 2

Heat a skillet over medium heat and grease with cooking spray. Pour 1/4 of the batter into the skillet; cook until bubbles start to form, about 2 minutes. Flip and cook until cooked through, about

1 minute. Transfer to a clean plate. Repeat with remaining batter.

Nutrition Facts

Per Serving: 362 calories; protein 16.9g; carbohydrates 7.4g; fat 30g; cholesterol 434.4mg; sodium 307.9mg.

Keto Diet Avocado Egg Bake

Keto designed egg and avocado breakfast for 1.

Ingredients

1 avocado, halved and pitted

2 eggs

¼ cup shredded Cheddar cheese

Salt and freshly ground black pepper to taste

1 tablespoon chopped fresh parsley, or to taste (Optional)

Directions

Step 1

Preheat the oven to 425 degrees F (220 degrees C).

Step 2

Scoop out a little of the avocado from where the pit was to make room for 1 egg. Place on a baking sheet and crack 1 egg on top of each avocado half.

Step 3

Bake in the preheated oven until egg is cooked, 15 to 20 minutes. Sprinkle Cheddar cheese on top and season with salt and pepper. Garnish with fresh parsley.

Nutrition Facts

Per Serving: 605 calories; protein 25.3g; carbohydrates 18.6g; fat 50.9g; cholesterol 408.2mg; sodium 525.4mg.

Vegetable Soup with Quinoa

This soup is made mostly of alkaline vegetables and is great for a detox. I crumble brown rice crackers on it before serving.

Ingredients

3 tablespoons olive oil

3 medium onions, chopped

2 green bell peppers, chopped

1 carrot, diced

1 stalk celery, diced

6 cloves garlic, minced

3 tablespoons ground cumin

1 teaspoon chili powder

1 (28 ounce) can crushed tomatoes

10 green chile peppers, seeded and minced

8 cups vegetable broth

1 (15 ounce) can chickpeas, drained

½ cup quinoa

Salt and ground black pepper to taste

1½ cups frozen corn, thawed

1 avocado - peeled, pitted, and diced

Directions

Step 1

Heat oil in a large stock pot over medium heat. Stir in onions, bell peppers, carrot, celery, garlic, cumin, and chili powder. Cook until vegetables are tender, about 10 minutes.

Step 2

Mix in crushed tomatoes and green chile peppers. Pour in broth, chickpeas, and quinoa. Season with salt and pepper. Bring to a boil; reduce heat to low and simmer for 30 minutes.

Step 3

Mix corn into the soup until heated through, about 5 minutes. Serve in bowls and top with avocado.

Cook's Note:

I prefer boxed organic vegetable stock.

Nutrition Facts

Per Serving: 253 calories; protein 7.8g; carbohydrates 39g; fat 9.3g; sodium 592mg.

Juicy Slow Cooker Chicken Breast For Any Diet

Super easy, low-fat, and low-calorie chicken breast. Great to set and forget on a busy day. You really can add just about anything to this recipe. I've tried everything from salsa to wine.

Ingredients

1 pound skinless, boneless chicken breast halves

1 (14.5 ounce) can petite diced tomatoes

¼ onion, chopped (Optional)

1 teaspoon Italian seasoning (Optional)

1 clove garlic, minced (Optional)

Directions

Step 1

Arrange chicken in a slow cooker. Pour tomatoes over chicken; add onion, Italian seasoning, and garlic.

Step 2

Cook on Low for 6 to 8 hours.

Cook's Note:

You can use any type of herb in place of the Italian seasoning.

Nutrition Facts

Per Serving: 144 calories; protein 23.1g; carbohydrates 5.2g; fat 2.4g; cholesterol 58.5mg; sodium 208mg.

Bulletproof Hot Chocolate

This is an alternative to Bulletproof coffee for people following the Bulletproof diet, ketogenic diet, or any high-fat low-carb diet.

Ingredients

11 fluid ounces hot water

2 tablespoons unsalted butter

1 tablespoon medium-chain triglyceride (MCT) oil

1 tablespoon cacao powder

1 tablespoon cacao butter

Teaspoon vanilla powder

6 drops liquid stevia or to taste

1 pinch salt

Directions

Step 1

Combine hot water, butter, MCT oil, cacao powder, cacao butter, vanilla powder, liquid stevia, and salt in a blender; blend until smooth.

Cook's Notes:

You can add 1 tablespoon hydrolyzed collagen protein powder and vitamin/supplement powders to the hot chocolate if desired.

I use grass-fed butter. Ghee can also be used in place of the butter, if desired.

Nutrition Facts

Per Serving: 478 calories; protein 3.1g; carbohydrates 9g; fat 50g; cholesterol 61.1mg; sodium 172.1mg.

Keto Vanilla-Cinnamon Cookies

Great cookie for a ketogenic diet.

Ingredients

1 cup almond flour

½ cup finely ground pecans

1 teaspoon cinnamon

½ teaspoon salt

¼ teaspoon ground nutmeg

½ cup butter

¼ cup erythritol

1 egg

1 teaspoon vanilla extract

½ cup coconut flour

Directions

Step 1

Combine almond flour and ground pecans in a skillet over medium heat and cook until golden and fragrant, 3 to 6 minutes. Remove from heat. Whisk cinnamon, salt, and nutmeg into the skillet. Set aside to cool.

Step 2

Combine butter and erythritol in a large bowl; beat using an electric mixer until smooth and creamy. Stir in egg and vanilla extract. Mix in almond flour mixture and coconut flour; stir until dough forms. Form into a roll, wrap in plastic wrap, and refrigerate for 1 hour.

Step 3

Preheat the oven to 350 degrees F (175 degrees C). Line a baking sheet with parchment paper.

Step 4

Cut dough roll into 24 cookies and place on the prepared baking sheet.

Step 5

Bake in the preheated oven until lightly browned, 12 to 15 minutes

Nutrition Facts

Per Serving: 92 calories; protein 1.9g; carbohydrates 5.4g; fat 8.2g; cholesterol 17.9mg; sodium 78.6mg.

Middle Eastern Tomato Salad

This salad is a perfect side dish for any phase of the South Beach Diet, or any other diet for that matter, and it's an incredible tasting summer treat for anyone, whether or not you're on a diet. I think it pairs wonderfully with any kind of grilled meat or fish.

Ingredients

1 cup seeded, finely diced cucumber

1 teaspoon salt

1 cup finely diced tomato

1 cup finely diced sweet onion (such as Vidalia)

1 cup finely chopped fresh parsley

¾ cup finely chopped mint, or to taste

2 tablespoons olive oil, or more to taste

1 tablespoon fresh lemon juice, or more to taste

Salt and ground black pepper to taste

Directions

Step 1

Place diced cucumber into a colander and sprinkle with 1 teaspoon salt or as needed; allow to drain for about 15 minutes. Toss drained cucumber with tomato, sweet onion, parsley, and mint. Drizzle salad with olive oil and fresh lemon juice and season with salt and black pepper. Serve immediately.

Nutrition Facts

Per Serving: 48 calories; protein 0.8g; carbohydrates 4.1g; fat 3.5g; sodium 297.3mg.

Eggless Pasta

Anyone on an eggless or low-cholesterol diet will appreciate this recipe.

Ingredients

2 cups semolina flour

½ teaspoon salt

½ cup warm water

Directions

Step 1

In a large bowl, mix flour and salt. Add warm water and stir to make a stiff dough. Increase water if dough seems too dry.

Step 2

Pat the dough into a ball and turn out onto a lightly floured surface. Knead for 10 to 15 minutes. Cover. Let dough rest for 20 minutes.

Step 3

Roll out dough using rolling pin or pasta machine. Work with a 1/4 of the dough at one time. Keep the rest covered, to prevent from drying out. Roll by hand to 1/16 of an inch thick. By machine, stop at the third to last setting.

Step 4

Cut pasta into desired shapes.

Step 5

Cook fresh noodles in boiling salted water for 3 to 5 minutes. Drain.

Nutrition Facts

Per Serving: 301 calories; protein 10.6g; carbohydrates 60.8g; fat 0.9g; sodium 292.4mg.

Chocolate-y Iced Mocha

My favorite morning drink that isn't a diet disaster.

Ingredients

1¼ cups cold coffee, divided

1 envelope low-calorie hot cocoa mix

Ice cubes, or as needed

½ cup unsweetened almond milk

2 tablespoons sugar-free chocolate syrup, or more to taste

Directions

Step 1

Heat 1/4 cup coffee in microwave in a mug until warmed, about 30 seconds. Stir cocoa mix into the coffee until dissolved.

Step 2

Fill a large glass with ice cubes. Pour 1 cup cold coffee and almond milk over the ice cubes; stir the cocoa mixture and chocolate syrup into the coffee and almond milk.

Nutrition Facts

Per Serving: 105 calories; protein 5.2g; carbohydrates 16.7g; fat 1.8g; cholesterol 2.9mg; sodium 255.3mg.

Low-Carb Beef Cabbage Stew

I modified another recipe on this site for South Beach Diet Phase 1. Not only is it on my diet, but it tastes delicious! Garnish each serving with sour cream.

Ingredients

2 pounds beef stew meat, trimmed and cut into 1-inch cubes

1 cube beef bouillon

1 cups hot chicken broth

2 large onions, coarsely chopped

1 teaspoon Greek seasoning

¼ teaspoon ground black pepper

2 bay leaves

1 (8 ounce) package shredded cabbage

5 stalks celery, sliced

1 (8 ounce) can whole plum tomatoes, coarsely chopped

1 (8 ounce) can tomato sauce

Salt to taste

Directions

Step 1

Cook and stir beef in a large saucepan or Dutch oven until browned, about 5 minutes; drain excess grease.

Step 2

Stir beef bouillon into chicken broth in a bowl until dissolved; add to beef.

Step 3

Mix onions, Greek seasoning, black pepper, and bay leaves into broth-beef mixture; cover saucepan and simmer until beef is tender, about 1 hour 15 minutes. Add cabbage and celery to broth-beef mixture; cover saucepan and simmer until celery is tender, about 30 minutes more.

Step 4

Stir plum tomatoes, tomato sauce, and salt into broth-beef mixture and simmer, uncovered, until stew is slightly thickened, 15 to 20 minutes. Remove and discard bay leaves before serving.

Cook's Note:

Beef broth can be substituted for the chicken broth.

Nutrition Facts

Per Serving: 372 calories; protein 31.8g; carbohydrates 9g; fat 22.7g; cholesterol 99.5mg; sodium 612.1mg.

Quinoa Dijon and Swiss Burger

Great dish for gluten free and vegetarian diet. Loaded with protein.

Ingredients

1½ cups cooked quinoa

2 tablespoons Dijon mustard

1 egg, beaten

1 clove garlic, minced

2 grinds fresh black pepper

½ cup chickpea (garbanzo bean) flour, or as needed

2 teaspoons vegetable oil, or as needed

2 slices Swiss cheese

Directions

Step 1

Mix quinoa, mustard, egg, garlic, and black pepper together in a bowl; add enough chickpea flour to hold mixture together to form 2 patties.

Step 2

Heat oil in a skillet over medium heat; cook patties in the hot oil until browned and cooked through, about 4 minutes per side. Add a Swiss cheese slice to each patty and warm until cheese melts, 2 to 3 minutes.

Nutrition Facts

Per Serving: 455 calories; protein 21.7g; carbohydrates 48.8g; fat 19.1g; cholesterol 119.1mg; sodium 474.8mg.

Instant Pot Vegan Potato Soup

Just because you choose a vegan diet, doesn't mean food have to be bland. This soup cooks in an Instant Pot, and is tasty even for those who have a normal diet.

Ingredients

1 tablespoon olive oil

Cup chopped shallots

5 cloves garlic, minced

1½ cups vegetable broth

3½ cups chopped potatoes

1¾ cups cashew milk

2 tablespoons flour

½ teaspoon salt

¼ teaspoon freshly ground black pepper

1/3 cup vegan French onion dip (such as Kite Hill)

2 ounces vegan soy cheddar cheese

2 tablespoons minced fresh chives

Directions

Step 1

Turn on a multi-functional pressure cooker (such as Instant Pot and select Saute function. Add oil and heat until hot. Add shallots and garlic and saute for 1 minute. Pour in vegetable broth and add potatoes. Cancel Saute mode. Close and lock the lid.

Step 2

Select high pressure according to manufacturer's instructions; set timer for 8 minutes. Allow 10 to 15 minutes for pressure to build.

Step 3

Release pressure using the natural-release method according to manufacturer's instructions, about 8 minutes. Unlock and remove the lid.

Step 4

Meanwhile, stir together cashew beverage and flour in a small microwave-safe bowl until no lumps remain. Microwave for 1 minute, stirring after 30 seconds. Stir into potato mixture. Use a potato masher to mash potatoes down to your preferred thickness. Season with salt and pepper.

Step 5

Mix in vegan French onion dip and stir until well combined. Ladle soup into 4 bowls and top with vegan Cheddar cheese and chives.

Nutrition Facts

Per Serving: 341 calories; protein 7.2g; carbohydrates 35.8g; fat 18.8g; sodium 920.2mg.

Low-Carb Taco Soup

If you are trying Atkins or another low-carb diet...this soup is awesome! This is a perfect recipe for a gluten-free diet as well. Easy to make and delicious. Garnish with cilantro and shredded Cheddar cheese.

Ingredients

3 cups chicken broth, divided

1 small head cauliflower, finely chopped

1 tablespoon olive oil, or as needed

1 onion, finely chopped

1 (4 ounce) can diced jalapeno peppers

1 pound ground beef

1 (8 ounce) package cream cheese, cubed

1 (26 ounce) container diced tomatoes

1 teaspoon ground paprika

Salt and ground black pepper to taste

Directions

Step 1

Combine 2 cups broth and cauliflower in a pot over medium-high heat. Bring to a boil. Reduce heat to medium-low; cook until tender, about 20 minutes.

Step 2

Heat oil in a skillet over medium-high heat. Saute onion and jalapenos until onions are translucent, about 5 minutes. Add beef; cook and stir until browned and crumbly, about 6 minutes.

Step 3

Transfer the cooked cauliflower to a blender and puree. Return to the pot; add cream cheese and remaining 1 cup broth. Cook and stir over medium heat until cream cheese is melted, about 3 minutes. Add the beef mixture, tomatoes, and paprika. Season with salt and pepper. Cook and stir until flavors blend, about 5 minutes.

Nutrition Facts

Per Serving: 377 calories; protein 18.4g; carbohydrates 12.6g; fat 27.6g; cholesterol 90.5mg; sodium 1281.5mg.

Cabbage, Leek, and Broccoli Soup

Just a nice, warming soup - great for diets! Garnish with parsley.

Ingredients

1 tablespoon olive oil

1 onion, thinly sliced

1 leek, thinly sliced

1 potato, cubed

½ cup broccoli florets

Cup shredded cabbage

2 cups vegetable broth

Salt and freshly ground black pepper to taste

Directions

Step 1

Heat oil in a saucepan over medium heat. Add onion and leek; cook and stir until translucent, about 5 minutes. Stir in potato, broccoli, and cabbage. Reduce heat to medium-low and cook, stirring occasionally, until softened, 3 to 5 minutes.

Step 2

Pour vegetable broth into the saucepan. Bring to a boil; reduce heat and simmer until vegetables are tender, about 15 minutes. Season with salt and pepper.

Nutrition Facts

Per Serving: 255 calories; protein 5.9g; carbohydrates 42.7g; fat 7.7g; sodium 567.2mg.

Vegan Sweet Potato Bread

Southern favorite that I modified for a vegan diet. This also freezes well.

Ingredients

1 cup chopped sweet potato

1½ cups white sugar

½ cup vegetable oil

1 over-ripe banana

1¾ cups sifted all-purpose flour

1 teaspoon baking soda

½ teaspoon ground cinnamon

½ teaspoon ground nutmeg

¼ teaspoon salt

 Teaspoon baking powder

 Cup water

½ cup chopped pecans

Directions

Step 1

Bring water to a boil in a large pot. Add sweet potatoes and cook until tender, 20 to 30 minutes; drain. Place sweet potatoes in a bowl and mash with a potato masher until smooth.

Step 2

Preheat oven to 350 degrees F (175 degrees C). Grease a 9x5-inch loaf pan.

Step 3

Stir sugar and oil together in a bowl until well mixed; beat in banana. Combine flour, baking soda, cinnamon, nutmeg, salt, and baking powder in a bowl. Alternate stirring the flour mixture and 1/3 cup water into the sugar mixture until combined. Mix in sweet potatoes and pecans; stir until batter is smooth. Pour batter into the prepared loaf pan.

Step 4

Bake in the preheated oven until top is golden brown, about 1 hour.

Cook's Notes:

Yams can be substituted for sweet potatoes, if desired.

The 9x5-inch loaf pan can be substituted with 2 small loaf pans.

Nutrition Facts

Per Serving: 295 calories; protein 2.6g; carbohydrates 44.2g; fat 12.7g; sodium 165.2mg.

Low-Carb Chicken and Mushroom Soup

Delicious restaurant quality soup for those on the ketogenic/low carb diet.

Ingredients

½ cup butter

1 cooked chicken breast, cubed

1 small white onion, finely chopped

3 cloves garlic, finely chopped

1½ pounds fresh mushrooms, sliced

3 cups chicken stock

3 tablespoons chopped fresh tarragon, divided

Salt and freshly ground black pepper to taste

2 cups heavy whipping cream

Directions

Step 1

Melt butter in a Dutch oven over medium-high heat. Add chicken; saute until lightly browned, about 3 minutes. Add onion and garlic; saute until softened, about 5 minutes. Stir in mushrooms; saute until tender, 5 to 10 minutes. Pour in chicken stock and 2 tablespoons tarragon; reduce heat to low. Season with salt. Cover and simmer soup until flavors are combined, about 25 minutes.

Step 2

Stir cream into the soup; cook until heated through but not boiling. Serve soup with pepper and the remaining tarragon on top.

Nutrition Facts

Per Serving: 531 calories; protein 15.3g; carbohydrates 8.2g; fat 50.2g; cholesterol 179.2mg; sodium 539.8mg.

Whole Wheat Oatmeal Strawberry Blueberry Muffins

I developed this recipe to add more fiber and develop a better diet.

Ingredients

1 cup whole wheat flour

1 cup oats

½ cup white sugar

2 teaspoons baking powder

½ teaspoon baking soda

½ teaspoon salt

1 cup milk

¼ cup vegetable oil

1 egg

1 teaspoon vanilla extract

2 cups diced strawberries

1 cup fresh blueberries

Directions

Step 1

Preheat oven to 425 degrees F (220 degrees C). Grease muffin cups or line with paper muffin liners.

Step 2

Mix flour, oats, sugar, baking powder, baking soda, and salt together in a bowl. Combine milk, vegetable oil, egg, and vanilla extract in a separate bowl.

Step 3

Stir milk mixture into flour mixture until batter is combined. Fold in strawberries and blueberries. Spoon batter into prepared muffin pan until full.

Step 4

Bake in preheated oven until a toothpick inserted into the center comes out clean, 18 to 22 minutes.

Nutrition Facts

Per Serving: 164 calories; protein 3.7g; carbohydrates 25.1g; fat 6.1g; cholesterol 15.3mg; sodium 245.4mg.

Baked Spinach and Egg White Muffins

These 'muffins' can be eaten warm or cold and are an Atkins Diet-friendly option.

Ingredients

cooking spray

2 tablespoons olive oil

2 cups fresh spinach, or to taste

12 egg whites

2 egg yolks

1 tablespoon grated Parmesan cheese

1 tablespoon shredded Mexican cheese blend

1 teaspoon garlic powder

¼ teaspoon sea salt

Directions

Step 1

Preheat oven to 350 degrees F (175 degrees C). Spray muffin cups with cooking spray.

Step 2

Heat olive oil in a skillet over medium heat; cook and stir spinach until wilted. Remove from heat and cool spinach. Squeeze spinach to remove excess moisture.

Step 3

Whisk egg whites and egg yolks together in a large bowl; add Parmesan cheese, Mexican cheese blend, garlic powder, sea salt, and spinach and mix well. Pour egg mixture into the muffin cups almost to the top. Place the muffin tin on a rimmed baking sheet and pour water halfway up the sides of the muffin tin to create a water bath.

Step 4

Bake in the preheated oven until muffins are set in the middle, 20 to 25 minutes.

Nutrition Facts

Per Serving: 108 calories; protein 9.4g; carbohydrates 1.5g; fat 7.2g; cholesterol 71.6mg; sodium 228.4mg.

Oven-Baked Beef Tagliata

This beef tagliata cooks in the oven and is perfect for those following a low-carb diet!

Ingredients

3 large cloves garlic, minced

2 teaspoons finely chopped fresh rosemary

1 teaspoon chopped fresh oregano

1 tablespoon sea salt, divided

2 teaspoons ground black pepper, divided

2 (1 1/2) pounds sirloin steaks, about 1 1/2-inches thick

1 tablespoon extra-virgin olive oil

6 cups loosely packed arugula

2 teaspoons extra virgin olive oil

1 teaspoon lemon juice

¼ lemon, sliced

2 ounces Parmesan cheese, shaved

Directions

Step 1

Place a cast-iron skillet in the oven and preheat the oven to 350 degrees F (175 degrees C).

Step 2

Combine garlic, rosemary, oregano, 1 1/2 teaspoons salt, and 1/2 teaspoon pepper in a small bowl. Rub spice mixture all over the steaks.

Step 3

Remove the skillet from the oven and add 1 tablespoon oil. Add steak and return to the preheated oven. Cook until steaks is browned on both sides, turning after 10 minutes, about 20 minutes total.

Step 4

Transfer steak to a cutting board and let rest for 10 minutes; then slice.

Step 5

Spread arugula on a platter and top with steak slices. Drizzle with 2 teaspoons olive oil and lemon juice and top with Parmesan cheese.

Nutrition Facts

Per Serving: 333 calories; protein 45.5g; carbohydrates 3g; fat 14.5g; cholesterol 86.3mg; sodium 1116.9mg.

Spiced Zucchini Carrot Muffins

Scrumptious spiced muffin recipe and a great way to sneak zucchini and carrot into your diet!

Ingredients

1 cup butter

1 cup white sugar

3 eggs

2 cups grated zucchini

1 cup grated carrots

3 teaspoons vanilla extract

3 cups all-purpose flour

2 teaspoons ground nutmeg

2 teaspoons ground cinnamon

1 teaspoon salt

1 teaspoon baking soda

¼ teaspoon baking powder

½ cup raisins (Optional)

½ cup chopped walnuts (Optional)

Directions

Step 1

Preheat the oven to 350 degrees F (175 degrees C). Grease two 12-cup muffin tins or line cups with paper liners.

Step 2

Combine butter, sugar, and eggs in a large bowl; beat with an electric mixer until creamy. Beat in zucchini, carrots, and vanilla extract.

Step 3

Combine flour, nutmeg, cinnamon, salt, baking soda, and baking powder in a separate bowl. Mix into the creamed butter mixture. Stir in raisins and walnuts. Pour batter into the greased muffin cups.

Step 4

Bake in the preheated oven until a toothpick inserted into the center comes out clean, about 17 minutes.

Substitute pumpkin pie spice for the nutmeg if preferred.

Nutrition Facts

Per Serving: 227 calories; protein 3.6g; carbohydrates 28g; fat 11.6g; cholesterol 49.8mg; sodium 254.4mg.

Tequila-Lime Chicken

This is an recipe that I created in search of a different way to fix chicken for a low-sodium diet.

Ingredients

3 skinless, boneless chicken breasts

½ cup tequila

1 lime, zested and juiced

¼ teaspoon garlic powder, divided

¼ teaspoon chili powder, divided

3 ounces shredded Mexican-style cheese blend

Directions

Step 1

Arrange chicken breasts in a baking dish; add tequila and juice of 1/2 a lime. Sprinkle 1/2 of the lime zest, 1/2 of the garlic powder, and 1/2 of the chili powder over the chicken. Cover dish with plastic wrap and marinate in the refrigerator for 30 minutes.

Step 2

Turn chicken breasts; sprinkle remaining lime juice, lime zest, garlic powder, and chili powder on top. Cover again and marinate in the refrigerator for another 30 minutes.

Step 3

Preheat the oven to 425 degrees F (220 degrees C). Uncover baking dish and discard tequila-lime marinade.

Step 4

Bake chicken in the preheated oven for 25 minutes. Sprinkle Mexican-style cheese over the chicken and continue to bake until the chicken is no longer pink in the center and the juices run clear, about 10 minutes more. An instant-read thermometer inserted into the center should read at least 165 degrees F (74 degrees C).

Editor's Note:

Nutrition data for this recipe includes the full amount of marinade ingredients. The actual amount of marinade consumed will vary.

Nutrition Facts

Per Serving: 244 calories; protein 22.5g; carbohydrates 1.7g; fat 8.8g; cholesterol 68.8mg; sodium 207mg.

Conclusion

The emphasis on fruits and vegetables that is at the core of alkaline diets offers the promise of healthy weight loss. No special gear or supplements are required. You will have the best success with it if you like to choose and experiment with new foods and love to cook. But following an alkaline diet will be tough for many people. A lot of favorite foods that are allowed in moderation in other plans (including lean meat, low-fat dairy, bread, and sweets) are forbidden here. Protein is limited to plant-based sources such as beans and tofu. This means you will have to make sure you get enough protein and calcium. Eating out also can be a challenge. If you travel a lot for work or have a busy schedule, you might feel bogged down by all the food selection and prep. Finally, many alkaline diets fail to address a major factor in weight loss and wellness success: exercise. You should include fitness in any healthy eating plan that you choose. The American Heart Association and the CDC recommend getting at least 150 minutes of exercise each week. If you have any medical problems or are out of shape, talk to your doctor first.

www.ingramcontent.com/pod-product-compliance
Lightning Source LLC
Chambersburg PA
CBHW050742260726
48661CB00001B/370